Qi Gong

8 Brocades

Qi Gong Lessons - Janine Isterling

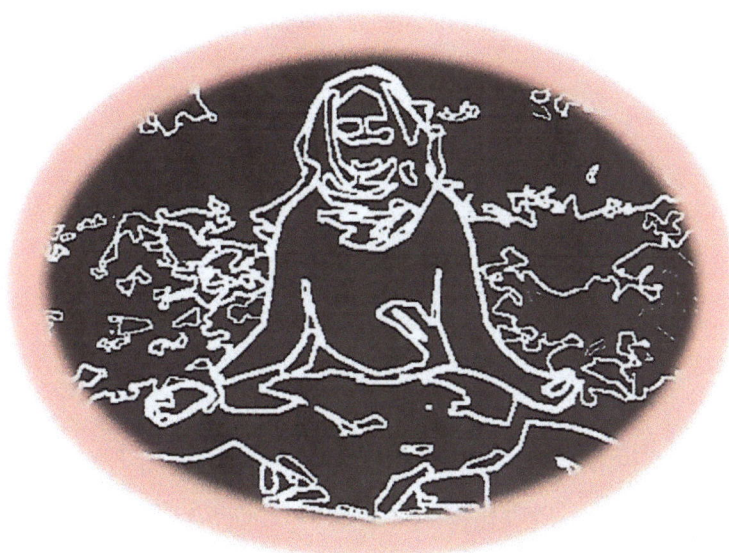

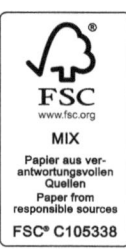
© 2022, Janine Isterling
Production and publishing: BoD - Books on Demand, Norderstedt
ISBN: 9783756202836

Contents

Qi Gong Lessons Janine Isterling – Time to relax

How I discovered Qi Gong

During my physical rehab at Foehr in 2010 I got in touch with Qi Gong. I participated in an exercise lesson and was totally excited right from the beginning. Back home I realized that for continuing with Qi Gong I needed professional help. But there were no suitable courses close to my hometown as Qi Gong then was not so popular and all relevant courses were completely booked out. So time went by and I was fully back in my daily routine and forgot about my plans. During the next time I kept on working in our open plan office. There I got tapped with laryngitis and two bronchitis plus various other infects. As I had been ill many times in 2015 I realized that something needed to be changed in view of my health and well-being.

I decided to do something for my immune system – and something for me. Thus I started searching and finally ended up with Qi Gong again. I found an article about Qi Gong and the 5 elements. I remembered my stay at Foehr and finally came to the conclusion to really give it a try this time. I had the chance to book courses but then I discovered the Qi Gong school in the internet. I had the decision between taking lessons or the education as a course instructor. I decided to mix business with pleasure and even get in touch with lots of theoretical know-how. I had interest in finding out what was behind Qi Gong and thus I made the move and signed up for the education as course instructor at Qi Gong School Bergstrasse. And never regretted this step ever since.

During my courses some attendants asked for a script and/or pictures which I finalized in an exercise description form. Also some adequate pictures could have been added with the cooperation of a friend.

Maybe all this can help to bring Qi Gong and especially the 8 brocades closer to all interested people.

.

General advices and exclusion of responsibility

Generally spoken, Qi Gong is not replacing a medical/doctor consultation. I as course instructor can never heal anyone or look into someone. Everyone who is not sure if Qi Gong is the right exercise for him should ask his doctor for advice. Also consult your doctor in advance when you are suffering from any disease, handicaps, pains or any health disorders.

When practising Qi Gong you do it on your own risk

The author is not responsible when exercises are practised falsely. The responsibility of the author is completely excluded.

In case of Yang symptoms such as high blood pressure, cramping, stress, physical fluctuations, hyperfunctions I address my attention to calm down, breathing out and relaxation.

In case of Yin symptoms such as depressions, weakness or subfunction I address my attention mostly on breathing in.

Never practise within the pain, only as close as possible to it. The exercise should in no case cause any pain.

Always pay attention to physical discomfort such as arthropathy, medical problems. In case of uncertainty always contact your doctor.

Do not practise in case you are suffering from mental disease (e.g. paranoia, depressions combined with hallucination etc.).

When suffering from heavy colds it is advisable to rather take a rest.
The exercises can be performed either while standing as well as while sitting down.

Basic Posture of Qi Gong

The QG basic position is the origin for all QG exercises and should be trained first. It is important to stand completely relaxed.

Situate your feet shoulder with apart and breathe in calm and softly in your stomach.

Leave room for breathing beneath the axilla also to give air to the heart meridian which begins there.

The palm of your hands point towards your body.

The feet stand firm on ground and are conceptually rooted with the floor. Your main focus should be on kidney 1 – the bubbling source – on the sole of your foot. That is the starting point of your kidney meridian.

The abdomen is relaxed and you slowly drop just like you would sit down while standing up.

The chin is easily edged upwards, the back is straight.

Inside your mouth you form the so called "Elsterbrücke" which means you put your tongue behind the upper incisors directing to the root of your mouth.

The shoulders are relaxed and stay loose.

Look forward and only concentrate on your breathing.

You can also address your view to the inside.

In your imagination your head is suspended like a puppet and drawn upwards with the help of the Baihui point situated in the middle of your head.

Conceptually concentrate on your position and create an inner smile.

I recognize my surroundings but without judging.
When starting with an exercise focus clearly and switch to the required position.

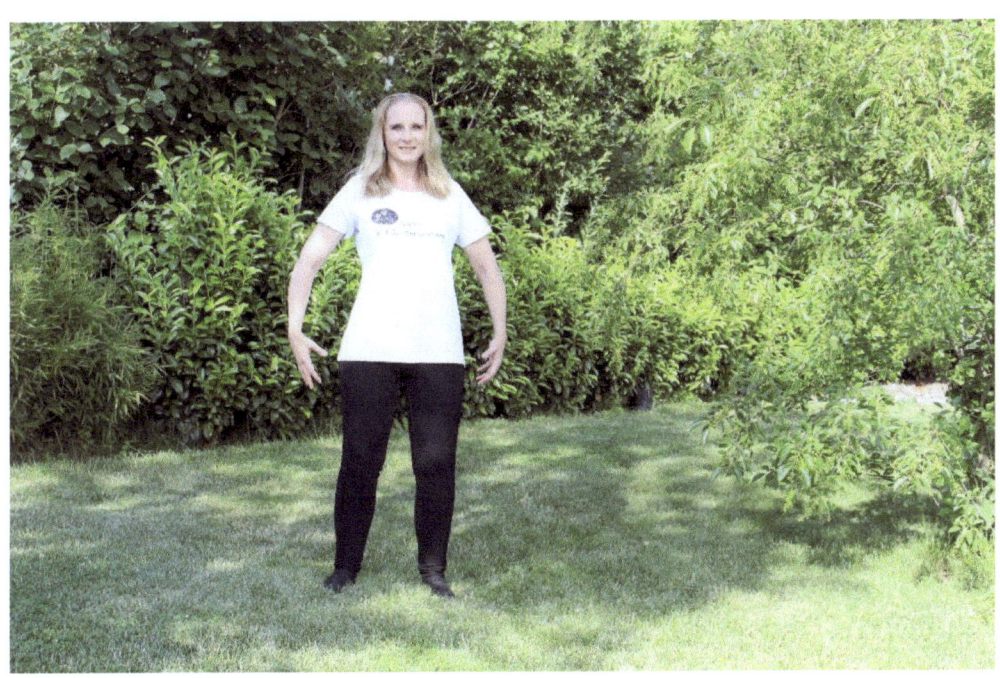

When exercising the 8 brocades we do not always stand in the basic position. We mostly stand upright with closed legs and not with feet shoulder width apart and arms beneath the body. We change position sometimes to a deep sitting or relocate your weight and move legs. Nevertheless most of the elements of the basic position should be kept clearly in mind. As the other elements of the basic position like pull up your chin, standing relaxed or even the concentrated breathing are still important.

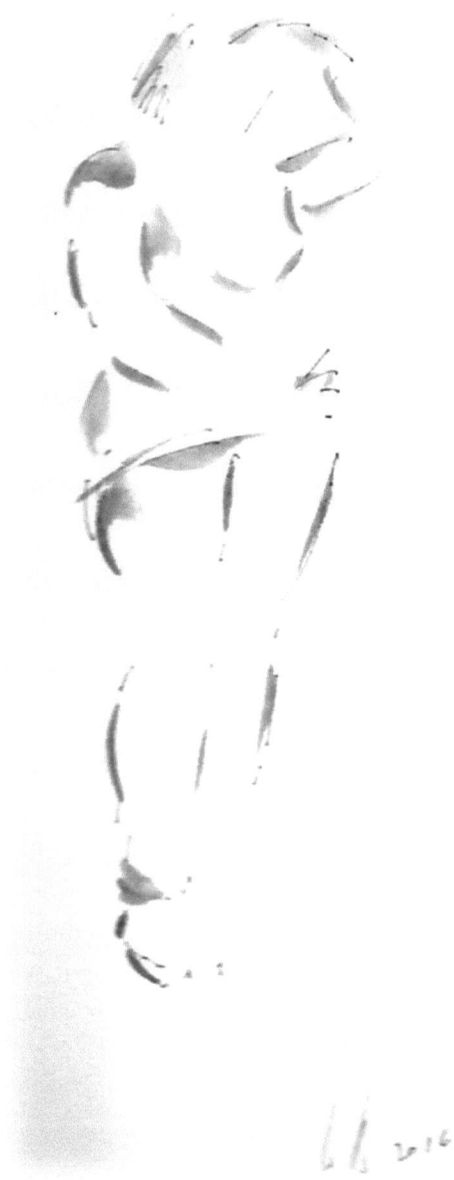

Qi Gong Lessons Janine Isterling – Time to relax

The inner smile

At the end of my lessons I like to include a small meditation or attentiveness practice.

Coming out of the silent Qi Gong there are two exercises which perfectly fit as follow-up to the 8 brocades.

One of these exercises is the inner smile. This exercise can be done either alone or as follow-up after the last exercise.

We either focus our view forward or look downward to the floor. It is important that nothing special is focussed. If you wish you can close your eyes. We slowly lower our eyelids. We sit, stand or lie down very calm. We recognize the noise around us but we do not judge it. We listen inside and only concentrate on ourselves. The breath is flowing soft and calm. After a certain time we take longer and deeper breaths. We welcome the relaxation. We send a warm feeling, a smile on the way through our body. We now guide this feeling as follows through our body:

- middle of the crown
- 3rd eye
- middle of the neck
- middle of the chest
- heart
- lungs
- liver (right)
- spleen, pancreas (left)
- kidneys
- finish in the lower Dantian (mid of your stomach)

We now slowly open the eyes, when closed, and see clearer and clearer

The small heavenly Cycle

For a better presentation of the small heavenly cycle I first of all established a chart of the human body from the back and the front.

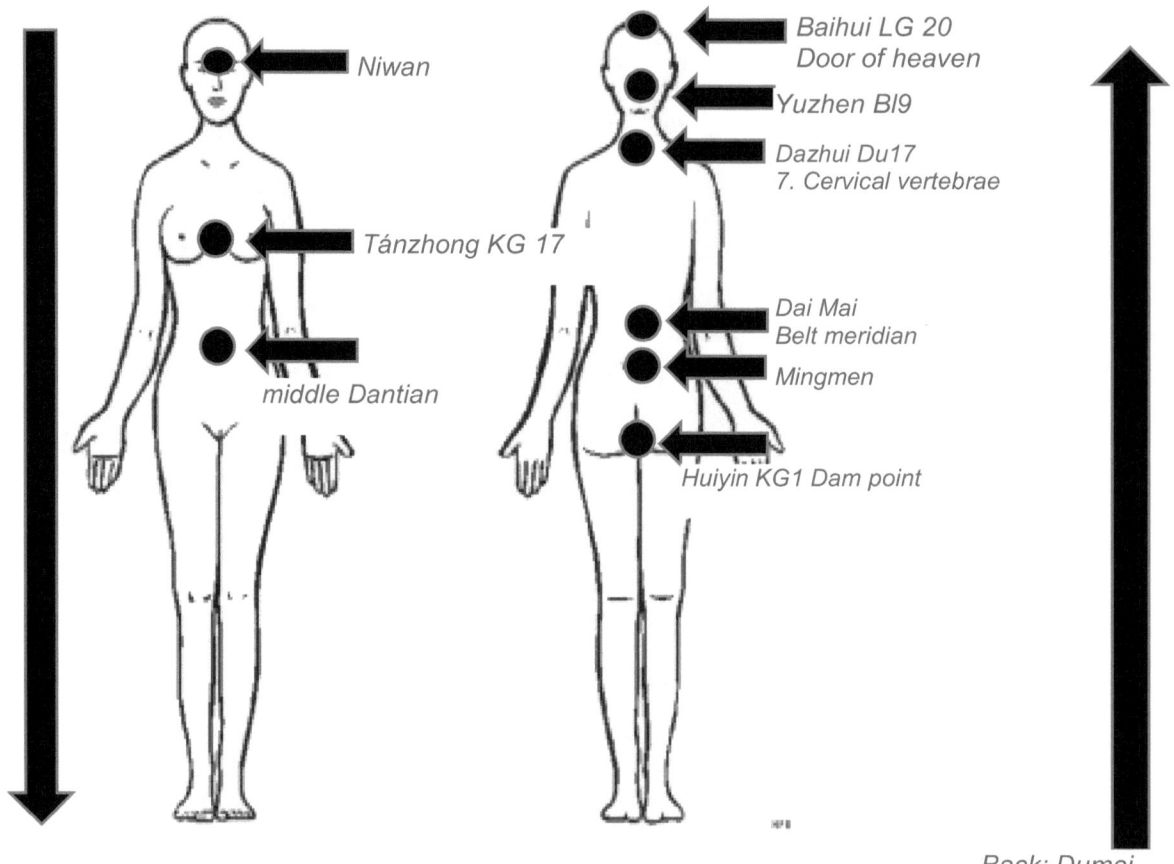

Front: Renmai –
servant vessel

Back: Dumai –
steering vessel

Qi Gong Lessons Janine Isterling – Time to relax

The small heavenly cycle is the second meditation resp. attentiveness exercise which I practise with my course participants. This exercise is mostly executed subsequent to the 18 movements either at the end of part 1 or separately.

I traverse the small heavenly cycle 3 times and thus bring my body in a calm, harmonized and relaxed state. The aim of this exercise is to draw the attention of the Qi to this stream. The exercise can be done either while standing or sitting down. I close my eyes and concentrate first to my lower Dantian (my lower energy focus in the lower abdomen). I rest my tongue at the roof of the mouth and close up with the „Elsterbrücke" the connection of upper and lower jaw and like that combine the Dumai and Renmai. The Dumai, the so called guiding vessel, runs up from the backside of the Huiyin point until the highest point of your head, called the Baihui point on your skull and from there it flows over the middle of your forehead to the roof of your mouth. The Renmai, the so called servant vessel also starts at the Huiyin point but it runs over the front up to your tongue. Without closing the Elsterbrücke there would be a gap and the flow would be interrupted. Reaching the Dazhui point I shortly rest and imagine how all pressure falls from me. Across the highest point, the Baihui point on the skull, I keep travelling forward across the Renmai down to the Dantian. Reaching the Baihui point I take a deep breath and when breathing out a healing sound of the liver – Schüüü – can be heard. When breathing out I inwardly sink down from the third eye – point Niwan – down to the lower Dantian.

In my imagination I let energy flow on my way and give my body strength.

This exercise always helps me very good if I cannot fall asleep. As I lie awake in my bed and my thoughts keep spinning around in my head it is most helpful for me to concentrate on the small heavenly cycle.

The 8 Brocades - Common hints and explanations

The 8 brocades are the most common form of Qi Gong.

The 8 brocades are also the „noble exercises". Their origin goes back to the 12th century.

People discovered records of Ba Duan Jin. The 8 brocade exercises are said to also be established with the help of Marshall Yue Fei.

These exercises strengthen our body, the breathening and our spirit. Thereby we rest our joints and effect a smooth stretching of our muscles.

The 8 brocades are usually done while standing. But also there is a modified sitting form.

The 8 brocades are similar also to the 18 movements part 1 suited for beginners.

In some exercises the hands are crosswise. Men put their right hand and women the left hand on top.

We always start the exercises to the left side.

In my opinion the 8 brocades can be executed all year long.

The warm-ups are usually the same, the final exercises, however, differ from the other QiGong forms.

YouTube Tutorials

Explanations to the warm-up exercisers, the 8 brocades and the final exercises can be found soon on my YouTube channel.

Just simply search for my name on Google and then switch to videos to reach my channel.

Between the exercises

Shortly rest („ground yourself") between the exercises.

Form a wide bow with your hands and rest on your lower abdomen, feel the effect. Afterwards breathe in 3 times through your nose and out through your mouth, striking out the belt meridian.

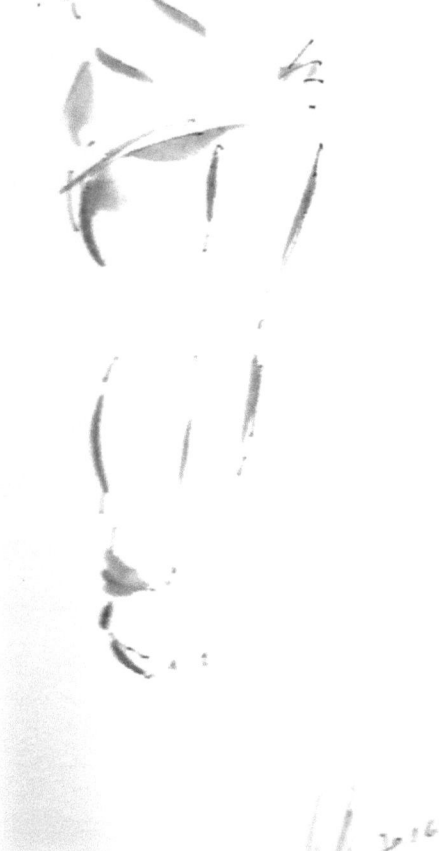

8 Brocades

1. Two hands raised to heaven
2. Drawing the bow to shoot the eagle
3. Separating heaven and earth
4. The wise owl looks backward
5. Shake the head & swing tail
6. Press the earth, Touch the sky
7. Punching with angry eyes
8. Lifting up the heels

1. Two Hands raised to Heaven

We stand shoulder with apart.

Our fingers are folded into each other in front of our lower abdomen (softly catching), the inside area of the hands show upwards and we lift them up to the middle of our breasts. Now we turn the folded hands towards our breast and move them all the way up.

Now our folded hands show outwards with the inside area and we lift them up our head. Our toes claw in the ground.

We look up to the sky (by making a giraffe neck), focus again on forward-facing and quickly release (flip) our fingers.

We lower our arms (joint by joint) edgewise and fold our hands again in front of the lower abdomen.

We stand solid at the bottom and loose at the top.

We altogether repeat this exercise 4 times.

Further hints to this exercise:
The three heatings meridian is a function and regulates for example the body temperature. It is selected in three parts and these support the body as follows:

-with the upper heater (head of your breast) we expand our lungs volume, we banish our tiredness and loosen our strain.
-with the middle heater (head of your stomach) we stimulate our digestion and encourage the organs such as spleen, liver, gall and stomach
- with the lower heater (head of your pelviabdominal) we stimulate our digestion.

We stretch our blood vessel and fascia

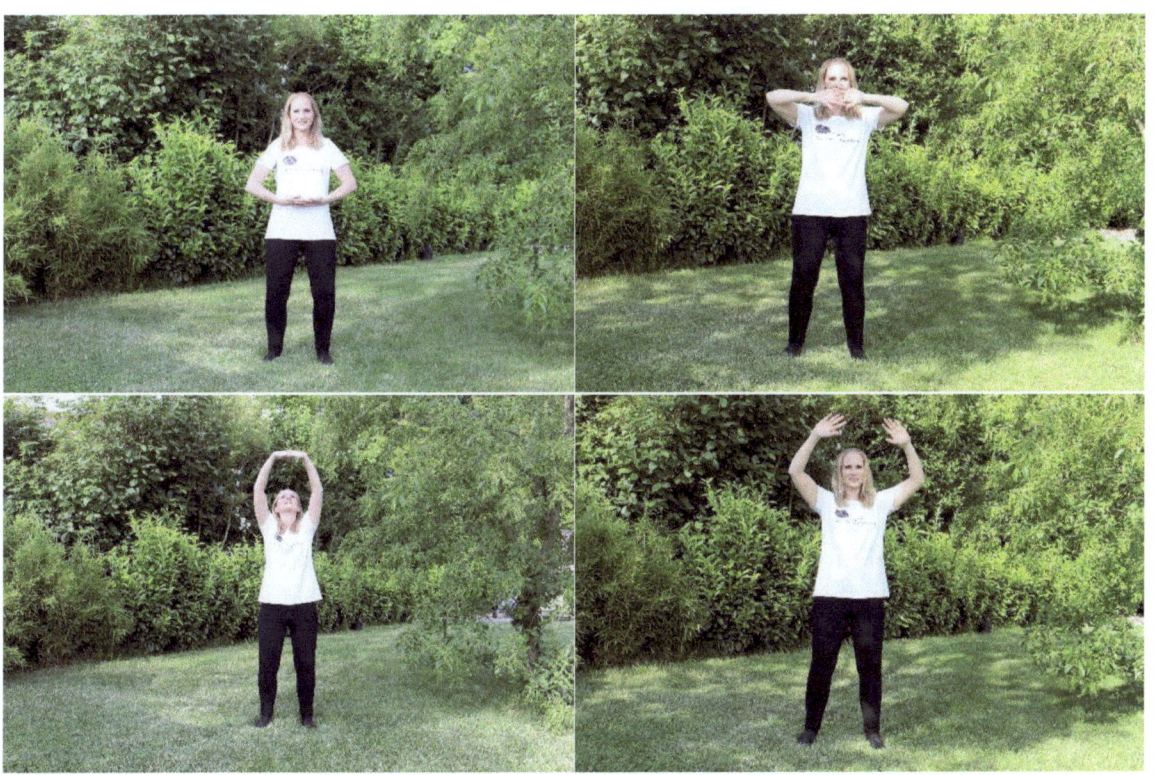

Qi Gong Lessons Janine Isterling – Time to relax

2. **Drawing the bow to shoot the eagle**

We stand with closed legs

We turn the right foot easily outward, cave in and open to the left. Both feet show slanted to the side.

We turn our hands, the palm of your hands show ahead and we lift up our arms sidewise using only our wrist up and down slightly.

The pulse move forward and we cross the wrist. At the same time put your left hand on top of the right one. Both wrists are pointing to your body. Form an arrow with the left hand, meaning thumb and forefinger are stretched like a V and the other three fingers are bent. With the right hand you build a hollow fist, meaning with the inside of your thumb you touch the outside of your forefinger (large intestine 1 to lung 1). The other fingers are bent.

We look to the left, turn the left hand (pulse on pulse) and your hands are pulled apart; meaning with the right side you pull the bowstring and put the thumb-forefinger connection lateral beneath your chest underneath your shoulder. With the left side we aim at the eagle and stretch out the arm to the left.

We open up both hands again, stretch out the arms lateral and stay long. We focus on facing-forward.

We lift up our body a bit, turn the right foot again forward and close-up to the right. Arms rest again sidelong your body.

Now we exercise the other side.

We repeat the exercise twice on each side.

Further hints to this exercise:

Helps against sleeplessness
Strengthen our cardiovascular system
Increase our concentration

Due to this solid stand we strengthen the kidney function

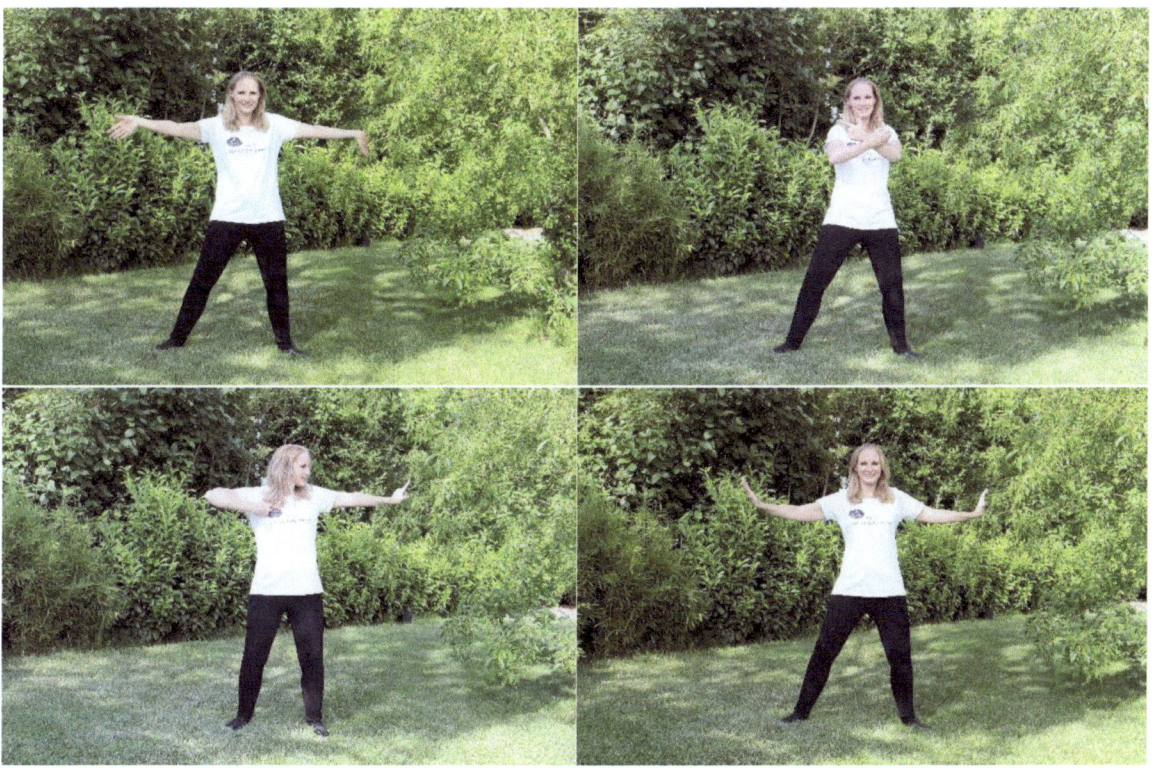

Qi Gong Lessons Janine Isterling – Time to relax

3. Separating Heaven and Earth

We stand upright with closed feet

Our hands are lateral beside our body and we lead them in front of our lower abdomen, the palm of our hands show down and the fingertips to each other.

We pull our elbows outwards. We lift our hands until the middle of our chest and turn the palm of our hands upwards towards our body with a slight rotary motion. We move our left hand with a slight rotary motion outward so that the left palm of this hand shows up. We turn the right hand down towards our body, the palm of this hand shows to the floor. We now support heaven with the left hand, meaning we direct above. The right hand supports the ground. We stretch ourselves and look to the right. Stretch both hands and relax, then we look forward, slightly sink in and simultaneously move your hands along your body back to your lower abdomen. The palm of your left hand shows downwards, the right one up.

Now we do this exercise to the right side.

We repeat this exercise twice to each side.

Further hints to this exercise:

We stretch the muscles of our back

We support our digestion (same effect as a massage) and regulate the energy of our stomach-spleen-circle).

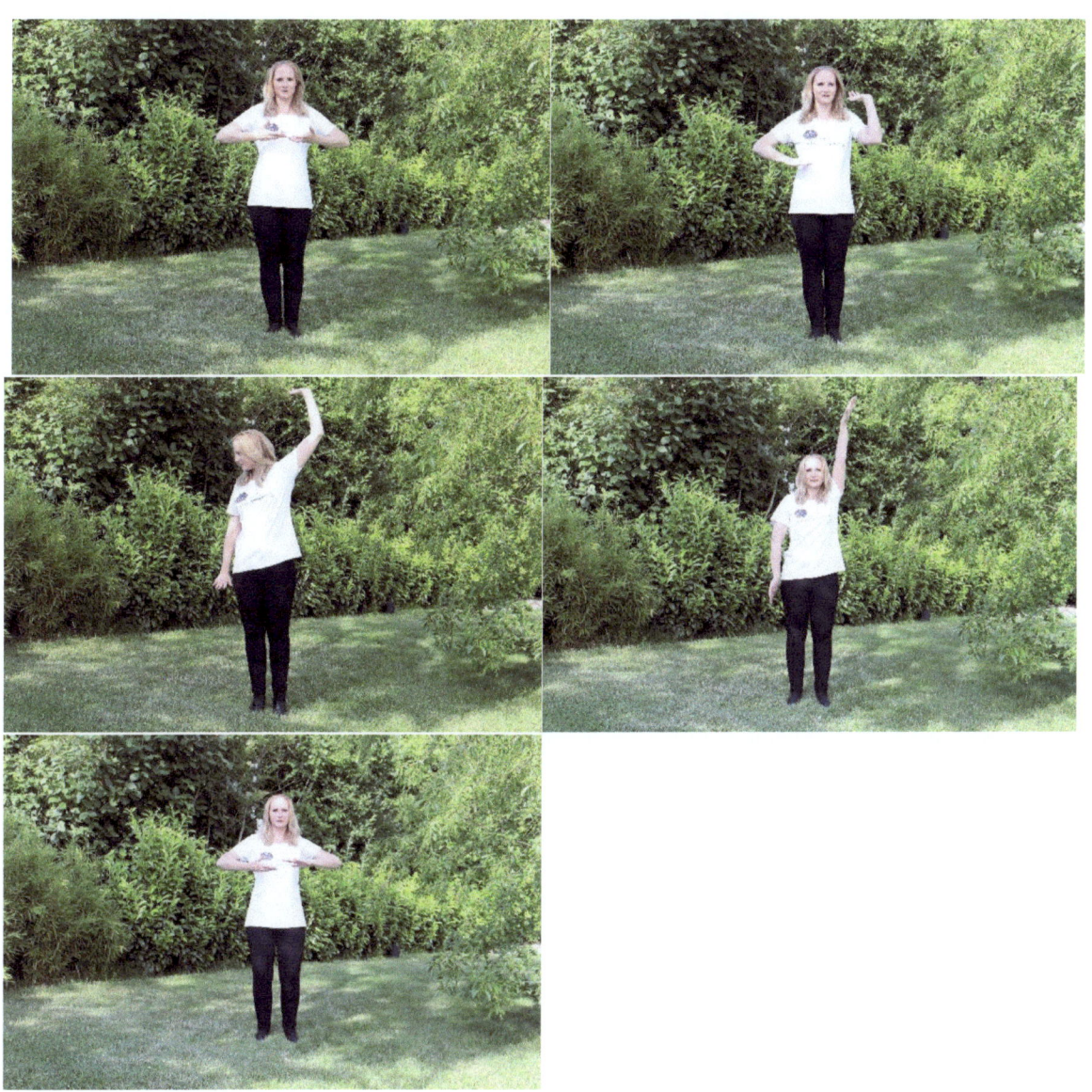

Qi Gong Lessons Janine Isterling – Time to relax

4. The Wise Owl looks Backward

We stand upright with closed legs.

Our arms are lateral on our body. We turn our arms such as the palm of our hands show down and lead our hands in front of our lower abdomen, the fingertips point to each other.

We turn our hands and lift our Qi on a level with our heart. We turn our hands again towards our body and let our Qi sink in our body.

We turn our head to the left, go up on the ball of our feet and turn our hands outward and to the back.

We look behind and let all being fall off.

We again turn our hands and look forward and once more sink in. The hands are again in front of our lower abdomen, the palm of our hands show downwards and the fingertips point to each other again.

We now exercise to the right side.

We repeat this exercise twice to each side.

Further hints to this exercise:

Strengthen the neck muscles and the eyes
The brain blood circulation is supported
We protect ourselves against the 7 emotions which are stressing us: Joy, anger, sorrow, grief, anxiety, fear and melancholia.

The 5 exaggerations which we drop are reflected in too much sitting down, sleeping, looking, walking or standing up.

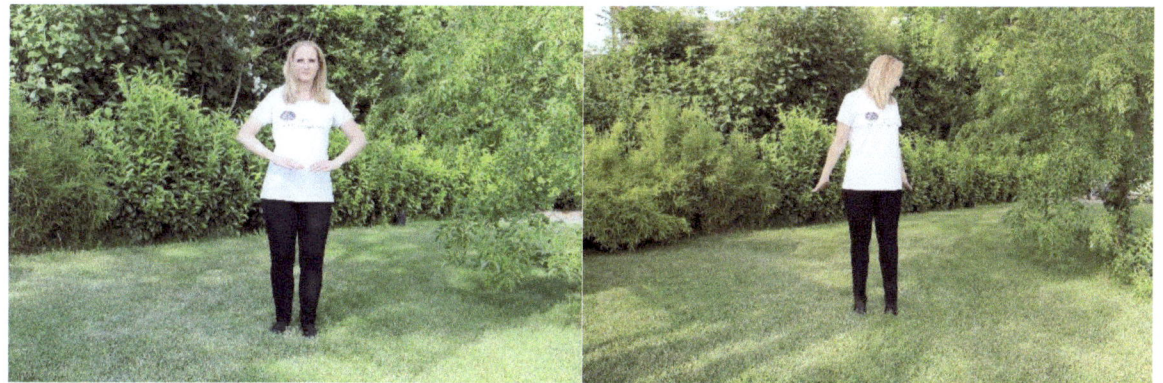

Qi Gong Lessons Janine Isterling – Time to relax

5. <u>Shake the head & swing tail</u>

We stand upright and open to the left in a wide stand.

We put our hands on our thighs, thumbs facing back, the other fingers overblown to the front and sweep down our thighs with pressure.

We relocate our weight on our left leg and look down to the right side facing our toehold. Our back is straight, not bend.

We move our upper part of the body as a bow across our front to the right side. Our weight is placed on our right foot and we look down to our left toehold.

We move our upper part of the body as a bow backwards to our middle and „sit" down. Now we are moving our bottom each 3 times to the left and to the right. Afterwards we push our breast/shoulder each 3 times to the right and to the left. Finally, but please real careful, we move our head to each side 3 times.

We lift up our hands and again sweep down our thoughts with pressure.

Now we exercise to the right side.

We repeat this exercise to each side twice.

<u>Further hints to this exercise:</u>

We support our abdominal area and can release hardenings.

This exercise feels relaxing, casting out your heart fire does not mean to cast out the love but to cast out the anger located in your heart. This is effected by the pressure of your hands on your thighs.

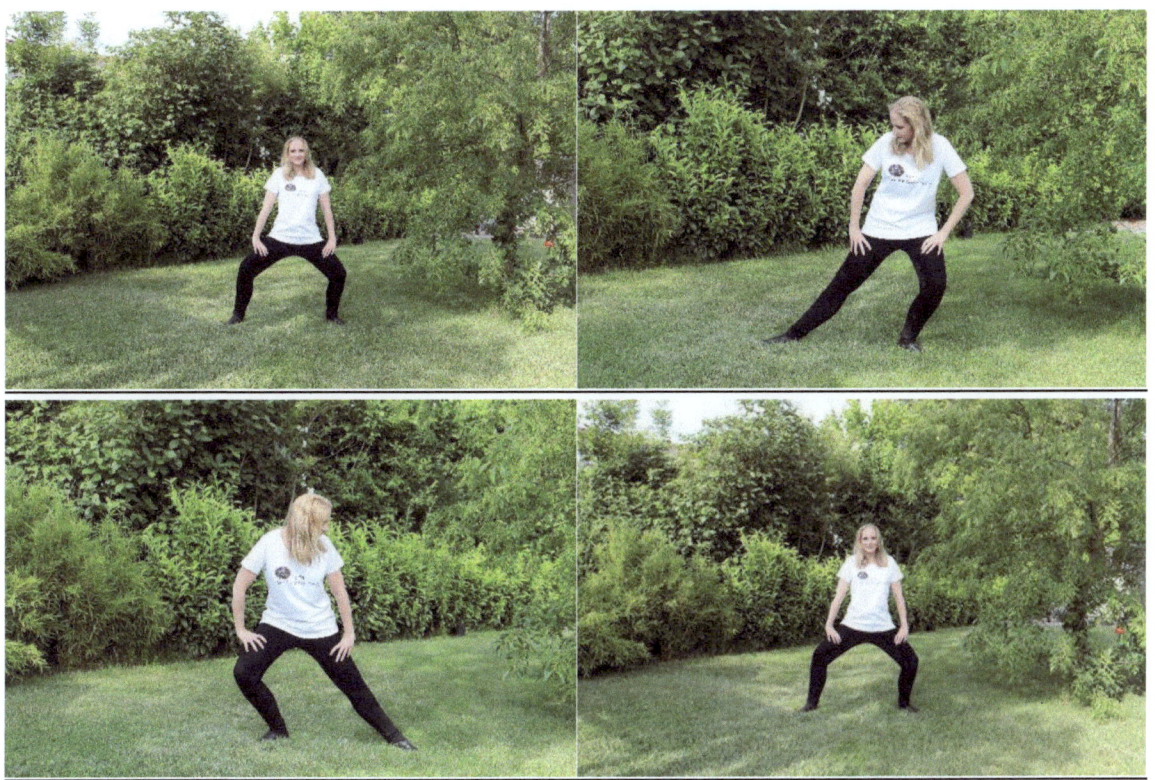

Qi Gong Lessons Janine Isterling – Time to relax

6. **Press the earth, Touch the sky**

We stand upright and shoulder with apart, our hands are lateral beside our body.

We laterally lift our hands, bringing the Qi up. We turn our hands, the inside area of the hands show downwards.
We lower our arms back down and let the Qi sink in our body. Our hands lie on our lower abdomen.
We open our hands towards the outside and sweep along our belt meridian, meaning with the thumb from stomach aside backward.

We put our balls of the thumb on our kidneys and push them short and gentle while we are sinking in. We do not put our head in the neck but pull our chin towards our breast, simply leaning back, pulling our pelvic floor closer and simply look upward. We again push our kidneys gently.

We raise again, bend down forward and sweep with the hands along the backside of the legs downwards, turn around the feet and sweep upwards along the inside, around the lumbar part up to the lower abdomen and sweep out the belt meridian again. Our hands are lateral beside our body again.

In case of troubles with the lumbar part you can bend your legs slightly. Apart from this we are standing straight when exercising.

We repeat this exercise 4 times.

Further hints to this exercise:

Very appropriate in case of low blood pressure.

We strengthen bladder and kidney function.

We promote the work of our midriff when breathing.

We stretch our body.

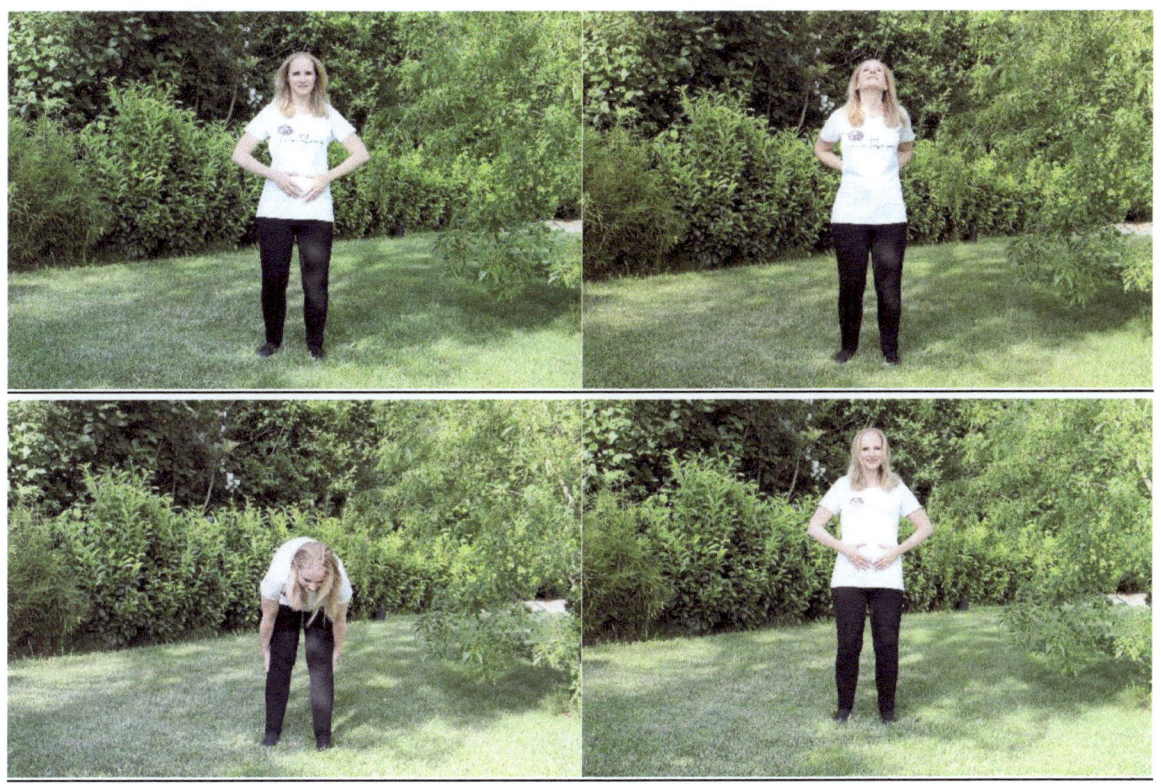

Qi Gong Lessons Janine Isterling – Time to relax

7. Punching with angry eyes

We stand with our feet solid on ground and slightly bend our knees.

We form fists beginning from our middlefinger and hold the fists lateral abreast our hips. We open our breast wide by pulling our arms (ellbows) backwards.

We take a deep breath and push our fists quickly frontwards. At the same time we widely open our eyes and call out loud „he". We breath out.

We now open our fists and the palm of our hands show outside. We again relax our eyes.

We pull back our hands again in spirals (first shoulder, then ellbows, then fist) and form a first again.

With this exercise we form a full feeling at the bottom and a really light one at the top.

We repeat this exercise 4 times to each side.

Further hints to this exercise:

Reduction of anger and aggression by screaming HE.

Strengthening your self-confidence.

The eyes belong to the liver and are being cherished there.

Improvement of the blood circulation

Opening of the upper respiratory system by pulling back of the arms.

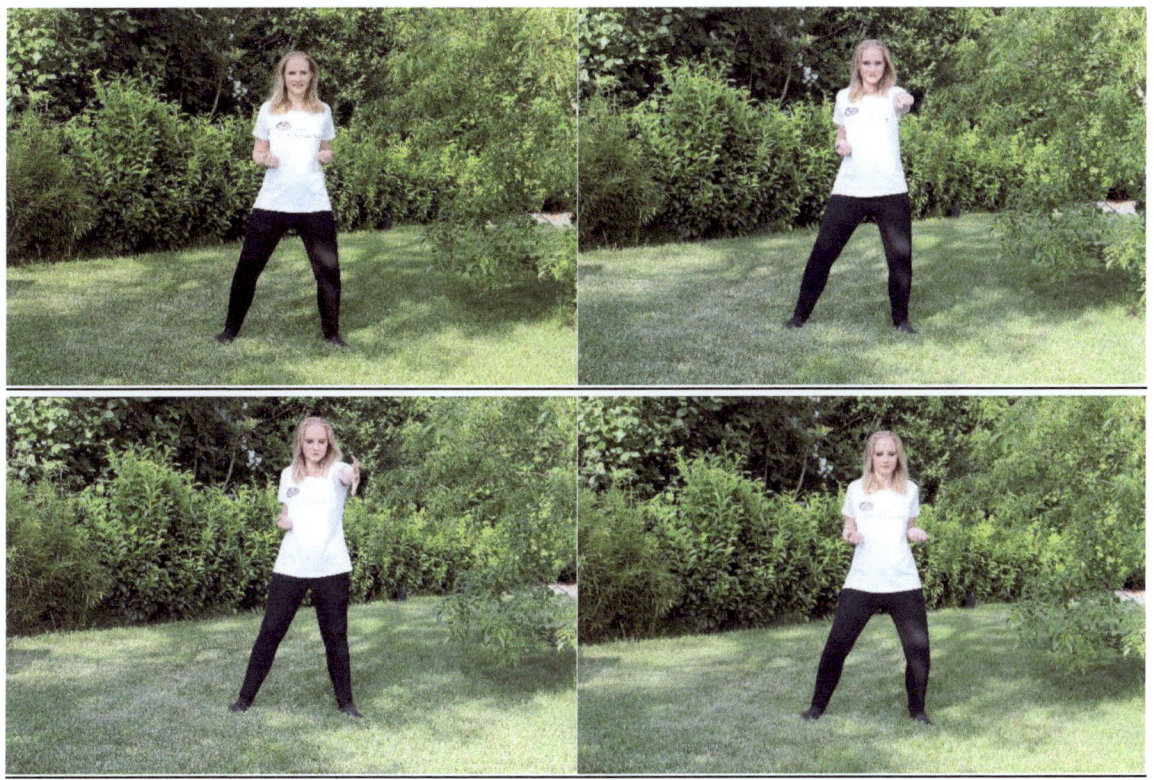

Qi Gong Lessons Janine Isterling – Time to relax

8. Lifting up the heels

We stand upright with legs closed.

Behind our body we surround one of our wrist with thumb and middlefinger of the other hand. Women surround the right wrist and men the left one. We put our hands as far as possible along our spine upwards. We stretch our body, take a deep breath and come down to our pad (the sparkling source).

We breathe out and let ourselves drop on our heels and at the same time let our hands drop to the Mingmen point (at the counterpart of our belly button in a straight line on our back).

We shortly wait and lift up our hands again and start once more from the beginning.

We repeat this exercise 7 times.

Further hints to this exercise:

We stretch and lengthen our whole body.

The blood circulation is stimulated by letting us drop, the Qi is flowing and we spread the energy through our whole body.

We can divert the wasted Qi over our feet as the effervescent spring.

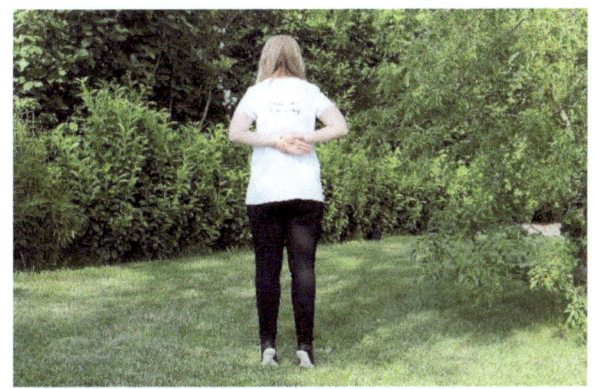

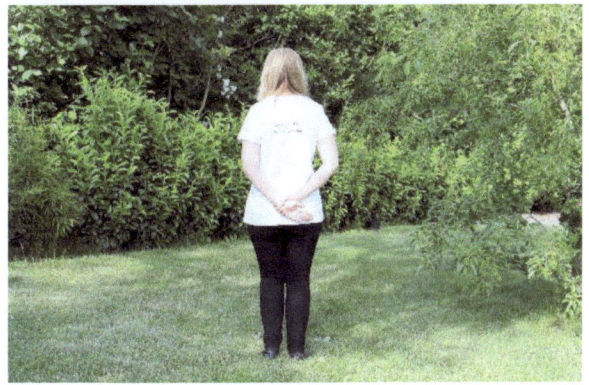

Qi Gong Lessons Janine Isterling – Time to relax

Thanksgiving

Special thanks to my kids A & Y for making me smiling every day and my mom for helping me to translate my book in English.

My special thanks go to my instructors Marita and Caterina Oriolo from the Qi Gong School Bergstasse. You have really taught me a lot and always have been very patient.

A big thank-you goes to Lothar Reker from Wyk at Foehr for his painted pictures showing me in „action". The original is in color but was redyed for this book in black and white.

Many thanks to Melanie for all the photographic work.

<u>Everyone holds his „Qi" in his own hands, so make something out of it.</u>

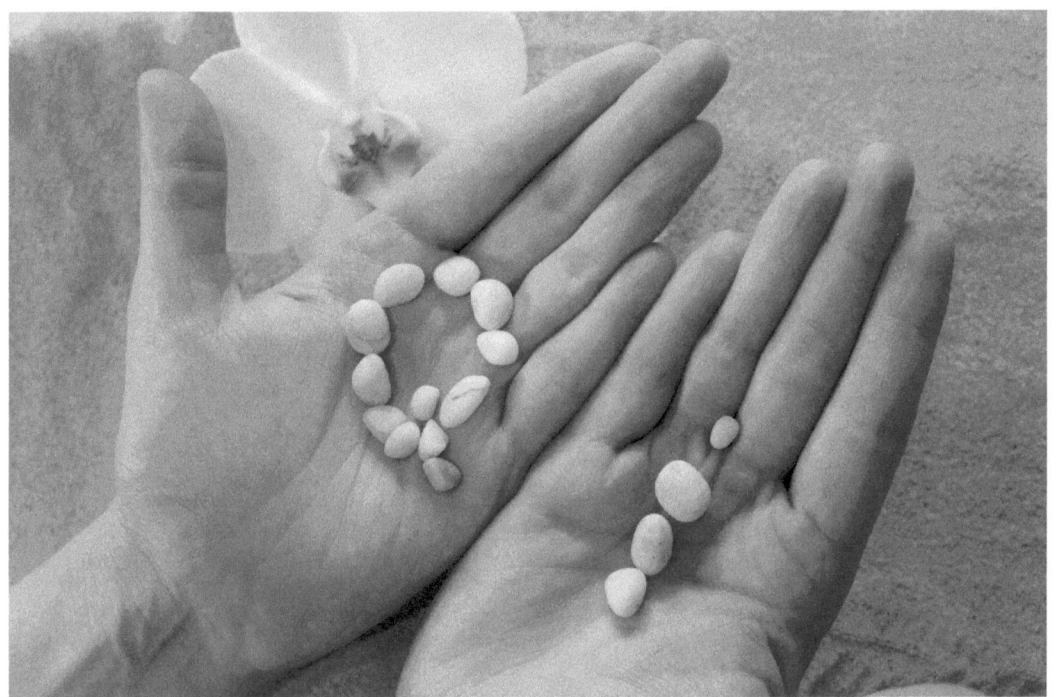

Qi Gong Lessons Janine Isterling – Time to relax

Îndication of sources and literature references.

As theory sources I have taken the following literature:

1. Wikipedia
1. www.gratis-malvorlagen.de
2. https://taiji-forum.de/
3. 64-schattenboxer.de
4. Abschlußarbeit Janine Isterling
5. Qi Gong Schule Bergstraße
6. Tai Chi Akademie
7. R. Wohlfahrt

All photos are in my full possession and show me in person.
All pictures, originator and usage rights are exlusively in my hands.
No copyprints, duplications, sales or exchanges of the photos are allowed.